The Aging Eye and Low Vision

A Study Guide for Physicians

D1276770

Editors:
Eleanor E. Faye, MD, FACS
Cynthia S. Stuen, DSW

Publisher:

THE LIGHTHOUSE INC.
1992

Barbara Silverstone, DSW
Executive Director

Harold Wilmerding
President

Acknowledgments

The development of this curriculum project began in 1987 when The Lighthouse National Center for Vision and Aging (NCVA) developed and offered a three-session minicourse on age-related vision loss to physicians participating in a geriatric fellowship program under the supervision of Judith C. Ahronheim, MD, at New York City's Bellevue Hospital. Former NCVA directors of education, Sydelle B. Levy, PhD, and Eva Friedlander, PhD, are gratefully acknowledged for their work on this curriculum. The Curriculum Advisory Committee, the chapter authors, and Rafael Sanchez, MD, deserve special thanks for their fine contributions.

The project support staff as follows is gratefully acknowledged.

Lois Gaeta: *Project Manager*
Juliana Wu: *Copy Editor*
Paula N. Dubrow: *Designer*
Ilene Linden: *Editorial Support*

Library
CORNELL UNIVERS

OCT 1 5 1993

Medical College
New York City

Copyright © 1992 by The Lighthouse Inc.
First edition.

All rights reserved. No part of this publication may be reproduced or transmitted in any form or by any means, including photocopying, recording, or by any information storage and retrieval system, without permission in writing from the Publisher.

Library of Congress Catalog Card No. 92-081854
ISBN 0-9603444-8-9
Printed in the United States of America.

Contents

Curriculum Advisory Committee

Carl R. Augusto
Executive Director
American Foundation for the Blind
New York, NY

Evan Calkins, MD
Coordinator of Geriatric Programs
Health Care Plan
Buffalo, NY

Jay M. Enoch, OD
Dean, School of Optometry
University of California
Berkeley, CA

Richard Ham, MD
Distinguished Chair in Geriatric Medicine
State University of New York
Syracuse, NY

Donald B. Maness, BS
Executive Administrator
Margaret Wagner House
Cleveland Heights, OH

Bernice Neugarten, PhD
Rothschild Distinguished Scholar
Center on Aging, Health and Society
The University of Chicago
Chicago, IL

Jay Portnow, MD
Clinical Professor of Rehabilitation Medicine
School of Medicine, Boston University
Westwood, MA

Rafael Sanchez, MD
Professor Emeritus
Department of Family Medicine
School of Medicine
East Carolina University
Greenville, NC

Jordan Tobin, MD
Director
Gerontology Research Center
National Institute on Aging
Baltimore, MD

Janet Townsend, MD
Residency Program in Social Medicine
Montefiore Medical Center
Bronx, NY

Stanley Wainapel, MD
Associate Director
Rehabilitation Medicine Department
St. Luke's-Roosevelt Hospital
New York, NY

Frank J. Weinstock, MD
Professor of Ophthalmology
College of Medicine
Northeastern Ohio Universities
Canton, OH

Ann G. Yurick, RN, PhD
School of Nursing
University of Pittsburgh
Pittsburgh, PA

The Lighthouse Inc.

Barbara Silverstone, DSW
Executive Director

Eleanor E. Faye, MD, FACS
Ophthalmological Director

Clare M. Hood, RN, MA
Senior Consultant

Cynthia S. Stuen, DSW
Director of Lighthouse National Center for Vision and Aging

Foreword

In 1954, in response to The Lighthouse commitment to individuals with low vision and some early experience with specialized optical techniques, Drs. Gerald Fonda and Alfred Kestenbaum began The Lighthouse Low Vision Service in one small room. Since the program began, we have experienced the gradual buildup of the momentum of the low-vision field until our message has been carried to 14 countries around the world and every state in the United States. Since 1975, we have offered low-vision courses to ophthalmologists, optometrists, nurses, and opticians as part of our Low Vision Continuing Education Program.

The contributors to this Guide and I invite you to join us in building our own special kind of momentum by incorporating the principles of primary low-vision care from this study guide into a plan of action in your everyday clinical practice. We look forward to being in close communication with you as our cooperative efforts enable more patients than ever before to make the journey from sight impairment to vision improvement.

Eleanor E. Faye, MD, FACS
Ophthalmological Director
The Lighthouse Inc.

Contributing Authors

Ann Burack-Weiss, DSW
Associate Professor
Columbia University School of
  Social Work
New York, NY

Norman Charles, MD
Clinical Professor of Ophthalmology
New York University Medical
  Center
New York, NY

Eleanor E. Faye, MD, FACS
Ophthalmological Director
The Lighthouse Inc.
New York, NY

Eva Friedlander, PhD
Former Director of Education
Lighthouse National Center for
  Vision and Aging
New York, NY

Clare M. Hood, RN, MA
Senior Consultant
The Lighthouse Inc.
New York, NY

Michael F. Marmor, MD
Professor and Chairman
Department of Ophthalmology
Stanford University Medical
  Center
Stanford, CA

Isadore Rossman, MD
Associate Professor
Albert Einstein College of
  Medicine
Bronx, NY

Karen R. Seidman, MPA
Director
Lighthouse Low Vision Continuing
Education Program
New York, NY

Cynthia S. Stuen, DSW
Director
Lighthouse National Center for
  Vision and Aging
New York, NY

Robert Sunberg, MEd
*Supervisor of Orientation and
  Mobility*
The Lighthouse Inc.
New York, NY

Rein Tideiksaar, PhD
Department of Geriatrics
The Mount Sinai Medical Center
New York, NY

William R. Wiener, PhD
Professor/Chairperson
Department of Blind
  Rehabilitation
Western Michigan University
Kalamazoo, MI

Introduction and Learning Objectives

The Call for Continuing Medical Education on Age-Related Vision Changes
by
Cynthia S. Stuen, DSW

One of the most rewarding aspects of the Low Vision Continuing Education Courses conducted by The Lighthouse Inc. has been the response of eye-care professionals to the ever-growing potential of treating age-related vision changes. As many of them have observed, "Years ago we wouldn't have seen these disorders because people weren't living so long." At the same time, physicians — including primary care physicians, ophthalmologists, internists, diabetologists, nephrologists, and others — are recognizing the interrelationship between eye function and hearing, visual impairment and neurological capacity, visual function and activities of daily living. They are learning how to improve the style and quality of practice management by incorporating clinically tested strategies and accommodations into everyday practice.

The goal of this independent study is to influence physician awareness of patients with age-related vision change, whether the change stems from the aging processes, chronic or acute disease, or accident. Particular attention is given to the educational requisites of the primary care physician.

Age-Related Eye Disorders and Their Prevalence

Older people constitute the most vulnerable group for such age-related eye disorders as cataracts, macular degeneration, glaucoma, and diabetic retinopathy. And, as more people live well into their 80s and 90s, both the numbers and percentage of older persons with vision impairment will increase. The National Center for Health Statistics (1984) reports that fully one-half of the visually impaired population is age 65 and over; some 3.3 million people have some trouble seeing or are legally blind in one or both eyes. This composite number includes 9.5 percent of the population between the ages of 65 to 74, 16 percent between ages 75 to 84, and 26 percent age 85 or over. The vast majority of these 3.3 million people are not blind and have some usable vision, often referred to as "low vision."

What Is
Low Vision?

Low vision is said to exist when ordinary glasses, contact lenses, medical treatment and/or surgery are unable to correct a person's sight to the normal range. The goal of low-vision services is to maximize the usable sight of a person to perform usual routine tasks, thus ameliorating functional disability.

Since vision is a complex sense made up of acuity, color sense, ability to distinguish contrasts, and evaluate the location of objects in space, low vision is manifest through impairments in the performance of any of these visual capacities.

Other age-related physical conditions may compound the effects of reduced visual ability and produce a more pronounced, but often unnecessary, functional limitation for older adults. Unfortunately, few physicians who work with older people are aware of the ways in which low-vision care can enable their patients to maximize usable sight.

While the main focus of attention is the over-65 patient population, the middle-age (and even younger) group needs constant surveillance. The harbingers of vision loss can first manifest themselves at any stage during the course of a chronic disease or can be a reflection of the process of aging. But there is another issue. Linked with the ever-increasing search for ways to match quality of life with quantity is the demand to contain spiraling health-care costs. Helping patients to remain functionally independent for as long as possible both to enhance the life experience and to keep costs down is a critical part of the overall picture.

Even so, nothing prepares a person for sight impairment. Reduced visual function at any stage in life has a profound influence on an individual's well-being. However, practitioners who are deeply involved in the specialty of low vision have witnessed first-hand that proper identification and evaluation of the low-vision patient enables the visually impaired person to forestall many of the potential sequelae. On a physical level, these might preclude accidents and falls.

The following learning objectives were developed after much consideration of the goals we need to meet.

Learning Objectives

Upon completion of this independent study guide, participating physicians should be able to:

- Actively identify age-related eye disorders and vision changes and perform a preliminary assessment of their effect on visual function of patients;

- Be able to differentiate between patients requiring acute care and low-vision rehabilitation;

- Assess the impact of low vision on activities of daily living and psychosocial well-being of individuals over the age of 65;

- Recognize possible visual loss related to side effects of medication commonly prescribed for systemic disorders;

- Mediate strategies for modifying the physical environment in the office, home, and outdoors to enhance patient care, as well as to help prevent falls and other untoward accidents; and

- Recommend and refer individuals with vision impairment to the facilities that have the range of adaptive devices and rehabilitation options that will help meet their needs.

This curriculum was designed under the supervision of a national advisory committee and this text was written by educators and physicians with a special interest in low vision. The Lighthouse Inc. through its Low Vision Continuing Education Program and its National Center for Vision and Aging have information and resource material available for professionals and consumers. Please feel free to call us at 800-334-5497.

Reference

National Center for Health Statistics and Havlik RJ. *Aging in the eighties: Impaired senses for sound and light in persons age 65 years and over.* Preliminary data from the Supplement on Aging to the National Health Interview Survey, United States, Jan.-June 1984. *Advance Data From Vital and Health Statistics.* No. 125. DHHS Pub. No. (PHS) 86-1250. Public Health Service. Hyattsville, MD, Sept. 19, 1986.

Chapter One

The Primary Care
Practitioner and
the Patient
with
Visual Impairment
by
Isadore Rossman, MD

A couple of years ago, after completing a general physical exam on a 75-year-old patient, I had a fairly serious discussion with him about his penchant for walking unaccompanied around the streets of New York. The reason was not the city's high crime rate, but the fact that his vision was impaired from both macular degeneration and early cataracts. I warned him that the streets and sidewalks of New York City can be an obstacle course, even for an elderly individual with good vision. I strongly recommended that he get a companion for his walks.

Whatever I said was neither persuasive nor intimidating enough. Shortly after, in the course of a morning walk, he fell through the open cellar doors of a restaurant and died from his injuries. By so doing, he became more than a statistic of falls in the elderly. To me, he is a perpetual reminder of the mandate for primary care physicians such as myself, ophthalmologists, health-care professionals, and family members to work together as a team to prevent such untoward events and to enhance the quality of life for those with age-related eye disorders and vision changes.

The mandate to be sensitive to the progressive impacts of age and disease is particularly critical for the primary care physician, who is in many ways the gatekeeper to care of the total patient. Whatever progress has been made in such areas as cardiovascular disease or infection control has been eminently applicable to the elderly population. It has been a major contribution to the phenomenal increase in the aging population, both its absolute number and as a percentage of the population. Unfortunately, this situation guarantees a rising rate of visual impairment.

The demographic revolution is illustrated in everyday clinical practice, where we see increasing numbers of the young-old (65-75) and old-old (75-85), and more and more in that rapidly growing sector, the oldest-old (over-85s). Their practitioners are given the first opportunity in identification of individuals with vision impairment

— be it related to diabetes mellitus, macular degeneration, hypertensive retinopathy, or cataracts. Timely referrals and close communication with the ophthalmologist concerning the patient's overall care can have a major impact on the functioning of the elderly individual.

At the same time, we must always be mindful that the challenges and opportunities for early detection and referral for treatment take constant vigilance. Many of the ocular manifestations of disease occur without symptoms. For example, small retinal hemorrhages, early proliferative diabetic retinopathy, or macular edema or glaucoma can be virtually as asymptomatic as the systemic settings in which they occur. Certainly, hypertension or unregulated diabetes often elicit no symptoms or complaints from patients. For these reasons, the primary practitioner should perform a routine ophthalmoscopic exam, ideally for all elderly patients, and out of necessity for all patients at risk.

I should like to clarify that I am not advocating that the primary care practitioner perform routine pupillary dilatation, a privilege that should be reserved for ophthalmologists. But I do recommend a reasonably diligent evaluation of the optic fundi and sufficient skill on the part of the primary care physician to recognize the important abnormalities. Since many of us are now equipped with lightweight ophthalmoscopes that we can clip on to the pocket of the gown next to the flashlight and the pen, we have this technology readily available. Thus, if the primary care physician and then the ophthalmologist both examine the fundus, we have provided the patient with two exams and better monitoring of early pathology.

Interaction Between Generalist and Ophthalmologist

Over my many decades of clinical practice, both I and my patients have repeatedly benefited from an interaction between generalists and specialists. In fact, I find that a telephone consultation with a specialist, such as an ophthalmologist, about a patient's findings provides a form of educational osmosis that is far more effective than standard CME courses.

Those of you who are participating in this CME study course

will benefit from the patient case studies in this text. For example, I referred to a retina specialist a hypertensive patient who had what I believed to be a punctate hemorrhage. After the ophthalmologic exam, which included fluorescein angiography, the specialist reported that the patient did not have a hemorrhage but a microaneurysm. He thought this might be the occasional microaneurysm found in some patients with hypertension. Also, he was certain it was not on a diabetic basis and that the retinas were otherwise entirely normal.

As a generalist, I always try to encourage the ophthalmologists to whom I refer patients to communicate fully with me about their findings — and their treatment regimens. As an example, the report that "there is no narrowing of the arterioles, no A-V nicking, and no evidence of hypertensive retinopathy" tells me that a patient's antihypertensive regime is successful. Such a report from the ophthalmologist might also lead the generalist to consider that the "hypertensive" patient may, in fact, have "white coat hypertension" or, possibly, pseudohypertension and that home monitoring of blood pressure by the patient may be indicated.

In many cases, to be forewarned is forearmed. Recently, I received a telephone call from a patient describing what appeared to be a migraine headache with unilateral pain and vomiting. When I checked his file, I read that he had a family history of glaucoma but not migraine and that the ophthalmologist had written me a note saying that the patient's intraocular pressure was somewhat elevated.

I was immediately able to make the presumptive (and correct) diagnosis that the patient was having an acute glaucomatous episode and sent him to his ophthalmologist for timely intervention.

Value of
House Calls

There are many ways for primary care physicians to get to know their patients. For example, as a primary care practitioner with a particular interest in the geriatric patient, I have made many thousands of house calls to patients. In fact, I consider these home visits the most rewarding aspect of my practice. If you want to get to know the total patient, make a home visit. By the same token, as my patients and their family members will attest, during the course of the visit, I am constantly alerting them to household risk factors and to safety measures that they can employ to help correct them.

As I have already noted, the problem of falls in the elderly is an around-the-clock threat.

Falls
in the
Elderly

Aging brings problems of balance and disequilibrium, with decreases in righting reflexes, increases in sway, and a terrifying increase in the number of falls. It is now clear that the chief risk factor for fracture of the femur in the elderly (both men and women) is the fall itself more than it is the osteoporosis. Impaired vision, of course, is a major risk factor.

To diminish the impact of postural hypotension, a cause of falls in the elderly, I curtail the use of long-acting benzodiazepines and phenothiazines at bedtime. To some of my patients' horror or dismay, I also recommend the use of bedside commodes, especially at nighttime.

An Approach
to Depressive
Reactions

The primary care practitioner is likely to have multiple opportunities to observe depressive reactions in patients to their visual impairment. Though not unexpected, the therapeutic opportunity should also be recognized, and depressive thinking should not be dismissed, especially in the context of overall geriatric decline. Specifically, when the impaired patient complains that life is hardly worth living anymore or shows increasing withdrawal, apathy, and giving up of former activities, we should entertain the possibility of a treatable depression.

There is increasing professional recognition of an entity termed "minor depression in the elderly." This entity falls far short of the better delineated and incapacitating major depression with its severe psychomotor retardation, vegetative signs, and weight loss.

Minor depression is easily overlooked, and it may be useful to elicit evidence for it by probing questions, such as: How do you feel about your visual loss? Has loss of reading ability had much effect on your life? How "down" do you feel? What do you enjoy?

What have you had to give up and how do you feel about it? How do you feel when you wake up in the morning?

Minor depression may be helped by the usual antidepressants. I have found small doses of methylphenidate of value. Major depressions should call for psychiatric consultation.

Even individuals who have never been formally religious tend to rethink their relationship with a higher power or being during time of illness and disability. Early in the evolvement of the Montefiore Hospital Home Care Program, I encountered members of the clergy who were making house calls on some of our patients. I was impressed by how positive an experience and how uplifting the visit had been for many of the patients. Therefore, the beneficial role of speaking with members of the clergy and patient attendance at a place of worship should be considered.

Support groups consisting of extended family members, long-time friends, and neighbors can provide welcomed aid and comfort, both in person and by long-distance telephoning.

Vision for the 21st Century

While the health-care delivery systems will redefine themselves into the 21st century, they will do so in the clinical setting of greater numbers of elderly patients with a predictable increase in significant visual impairments. To treat these patients effectively, we must anticipate and prevent wherever possible, and encourage ongoing communication between all members of the health-care team and patient's support group. Clearly, the primary care practitioner will remain in the forefront and will carry out the most basic and ongoing role. With regard to age-related vision changes and disorders, the challenge, as always, begins with early recognition.

Chapter Two

Normal Age-Related
Vision Changes
and
Their Effects
on Vision
by
Michael F. Marmor, MD

It is debatable whether any decline in visual function with age is truly "normal," or whether the process of aging is strictly necessary. This argument is beyond our scope, however, and will be avoided by simply describing the quality of vision that is found typically in older individuals. However, it is still necessary to distinguish between a quality of vision that we accept as an accompaniment of good health and that which we call pathologic because it impairs ordinary levels of function. Definite changes occur in vision with age, but, in general, excellent visual function is the rule rather than the exception. Poor vision among older adults should be medically evaluated, and never just passed off as a function of age.

Anatomic Changes

Many of the visual effects of age are a direct result of anatomic changes that characterize the older eye. The cornea generally remains clear in old age, but as some of the endothelial cells (which maintain thinness and clarity) drop out, the cornea may become slightly thicker and more likely to scatter light. The lens invariably becomes more dense, more yellow, and less elastic, and these changes account for some of the subtle visual changes as well as the loss of accommodation. The pupil becomes smaller with age, so that less light is admitted to the eye and there is less capacity to adjust to changing levels of illumination. The vitreous gel tends to condense and collapse, and bits of dense gel may be visible as floaters against a sky or white wall. The retinal vasculature ages along with vasculature elsewhere in the body. Finally, the retina is embryonically a part of the brain that loses cells, and a gradual loss of nerve cells within the retina and visual cortex occurs over the years.

Examples of Age-Related Vision Changes

■ **Cornea** — Generally remains clear. However, some of the endothelial cells (which maintain thinness and clarity) drop out. As a result, the cornea might become slightly thicker and more likely to scatter light.

■ **Lens** — Invariably becomes denser, more yellow, and less elastic. These changes account for subtle visual changes, as well as the loss of accommodation (focusing power).

■ **Pupil** — Generally becomes smaller, permitting less light to be admitted to the eye. The individual has less capacity to adjust to changing levels of illumination.

■ **Vitreous gel** — Tends to condense and collapse. Bits of dense gel may appear as floaters against the sky or a white wall.

■ **Retina** — Embryonically a part of the brain (which loses cells). The number of nerve cells within the retina and visual cortex gradually reduce over time.

■ **Retinal vasculature** — Ages along with vasculature throughout the body.

Visual Acuity

The Framingham Heart Study, based upon prospective examination of an entire town, showed that visual acuity is remarkably well preserved in the elderly population. Corrected visual acuity of at least 20/25 in the better eye is retained by 98 percent of individuals between ages 52 and 64, 92 percent between 65 and 74, and 70 percent between 75 and 85. Furthermore, 87 percent of this latter group had visual acuity of 20/40 or better. Thus, we should not expect poor acuity in the elderly. At the same time, these data show that more than 10 percent of the population over 75 has acuity poor enough to affect driving and other day-to-day tasks. A significant minority of elderly patients have pathologic visual impairment that needs to be recognized in order to receive medical treatment and advice on managing their disability.

The causes of diminished visual acuity with age are not entirely clear. A good part of the loss undoubtedly results from aging changes in the lens, narrowing of the pupil, and the gradual loss of visual neurons. The fact that a few elderly individuals retain exceptionally sharp acuity gives hope that the aging process might eventually be moderated.

Accommodation

Perhaps the most universal age-related ocular deficiency is presbyopia, or the loss of accommodation (focusing power). A young child can hold print practically up to the nose, but somewhere between ages 45 and 50, individuals corrected for distance vision will start holding the newspaper at arm's length. By roughly age 60, accommodation stabilizes at a low level, and virtually everyone must wear different glasses for reading than for distance. Note that presbyopia is solely a matter of focusing power, and has nothing to do with basic nearsightedness or farsightedness (which describe the overall optical configuration of the eye).

Presbyopia is mostly a nuisance, since optical correction is easily available as bifocals, trifocals, reading glasses or continuous-range glasses. It may cause difficulty in certain situations, however. For example, individuals wearing bifocals have difficulty walking down the stairs since they cannot see their feet through the reading segment. Bifocals are also ill-suited for intermediate-distance tasks, such as playing music or using a computer. Special glasses may be worth the cost to facilitate these activities.

Color
and
Night
Vision

It is unclear whether color vision or night vision are intrinsically diminished in the elderly, or are simply affected by the changes in the pupil and the lens. Regardless, most elderly individuals adjust more slowly to changes in illumination and, even when fully dark-adapted, are unable to see in quite dim a light as a youthful observer. The latter problem is not of much concern, since in our lighted world we rarely function at maximum sensitivity. However, the sluggishness of adjustment can be most annoying going in and out of sunlight, or going into a dark theater or restaurant. Many older individuals find that blues appear dark and hard to distinguish from greens, presumably because the yellowish elderly lens absorbs blue light selectively. After cataract surgery, most patients will notice a brightening of colors at the blue end of the spectrum.

Contrast and Glare Sensitivity

Visual acuity is important for reading, but the recognition of objects and faces in the real world requires the recognition of contrasts, textures, and patterns. Most of the cells in our retina and brain are coded to recognize edges and contrast, rather than absolute light or darkness. Thus, our ability to discriminate light from dark is central to the process of perception. Even older individuals with excellent visual acuity usually have some loss of contrast sensitivity, meaning that they need sharper contrasts and sharper edges to discriminate objects than would a younger person. Much of this loss probably relates to the reduced light admitted through the small pupil and the increased density or haziness of the older lens. The net effect is that it is harder to recognize faces and objects, especially at dusk or in dim lighting where contrast is poor.

These difficulties are made worse by increased sensitivity to glare. Since even minimal haze in the cornea or lens will scatter light and interfere with vision, older individuals are often susceptible to discomfort and sometimes even disability under bright outdoor conditions, and when facing such bright sources of light as oncoming headlights.

Patient Education for Bifocal Wearers

- Take care when walking down stairs or steep inclines. Feet cannot be seen through the reading segment.
- Standard bifocals may not be effective for playing music or working at a computer.
- Trifocal-lens glasses, or separate intermediate-distance glasses, may be worth the cost to facilitate these activities.

Visual Quality and Illumination

To the extent that we can characterize "normal" vision in older adults, it might be said that acuity remains fairly sharp, but the quality of vision is not what it used to be. When lighting is optimal and the subject is sharply defined (such as black print on a white page), vision is quite good. But vision is more difficult under conditions of adverse lighting or changing illumination, and subtle contrasts or colors might be difficult to discriminate. For these reasons, environmental conditions and lighting are much more critical to the elderly than to the young. Harsh or "cold" lighting may cause glare and discomfort. In contrast, indirect and warm (incandescent) lighting is apt to be more comfortable. Glare from the sun outdoors or from an unfortunately placed window can be very distracting. Dim indoor lighting or lightly colored signs and labels will be very difficult to see. Thus, paradoxically, older individuals need more light to see, and are also more sensitive to interference and glare.

Outdoors, the use of good sunglasses, either a neutral gray to reduce light intensity or yellow-orange or amber lenses that absorb at the blue end of the spectrum, can reduce glare and enhance both comfort and contrast sensitivity. Occasionally, the indoor use of yellowish or amber filters may be helpful. The bottom line is that the quality of vision, although difficult to test in the office, is a valid and important parameter for daily life. If complaints about the quality of vision are taken seriously, many of the problems can be minimized with knowledgeable advice and common sense.

Advice on Lighting and Glare

■ "Warm" incandescent lighting is often more comfortable than "cold" fluorescent lighting.

■ Sunglasses that block all ultraviolet light (and even some blue light) may increase comfort and minimize stress on the retina. A wide-brimmed hat provides added protection.

■ Individuals who are especially sensitive to glare or poor contrast may get some relief from yellow or amber lenses.

Chapter Three

Age-Related
Eye Diseases and
Their Effects on
Visual Function
by
Michael F. Marmor, MD

Although the quality of vision may diminish in subtle ways with age, visual acuity often remains excellent. Difficulty in reading, driving, recognizing friends, or walking in unfamiliar territory are signs of abnormality — and they should not be excused on the basis of "old age." A relatively small list of diseases accounts for the majority of geriatric visual problems. Most of these diseases can be recognized by the general physician with minimal diagnostic testing and equipment, and early diagnosis can prevent irreversible visual loss.

It is difficult to assess the retina and optic nerve without dilating the pupil, especially in older patients in whom the pupil is small and the lens mildly cataractous. In the majority of patients, it is safe to dilate the pupils, and you gain a much better view inside the eye, for medical as well as ophthalmologic purposes. The only significant risk is that of narrow-angle glaucoma, which is relatively rare and occurs only in eyes that are predisposed by a shallow anterior chamber (see section on glaucoma for notes on how to judge anterior chamber depth). For routine pupillary dilatations, I recommend tropicamide, a short-acting anticholinergic agent that lasts only 1 to 2 hours. One may also use 2.5% phenylephrine, but it lasts longer and may have a systemic pressor effect.

Cataracts

Mild yellowing and cloudiness of the lens is almost universal in older individuals, but a cataract is not "visually significant" until it impairs function at a level that bothers the patient. There is virtually no reason to remove cataracts "because they are there." Patients with cataract complain of poor visual acuity, difficulty seeing under dim light, and increased sensitivity to glare. Cataracts can usually be recognized with a direct ophthalmoscope. With a high "plus" setting, you normally see a bright red reflection through the pupil as you approach the eye. If there is a

The Eye:
Its visible and internal structures

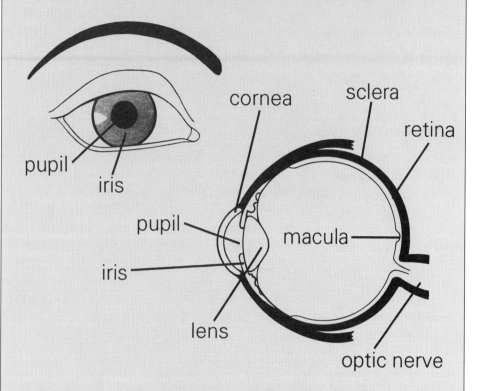

pupil

iris

cornea

sclera

retina

pupil

iris

macula

lens

optic nerve

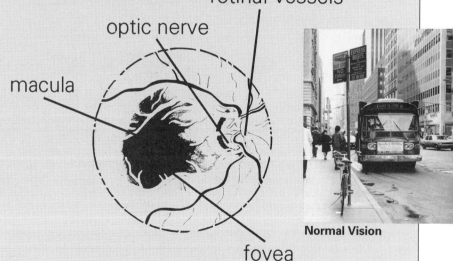

retinal vessels

optic nerve

macula

fovea

Normal Vision

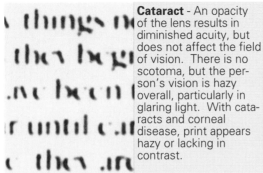

Cataract - An opacity of the lens results in diminished acuity, but does not affect the field of vision. There is no scotoma, but the person's vision is hazy overall, particularly in glaring light. With cataracts and corneal disease, print appears hazy or lacking in contrast.

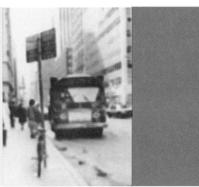

dark shadow in the midst of the red reflex, or the pupil remains dark, cataract is a likely cause.

Cataract surgery is highly successful: 95 percent of patients have significantly improved vision unless there is underlying retinal or optic nerve damage. Most older patients nowadays have implantation of an intraocular lens, thereby eliminating the need for thick spectacles or a contact lens. Several techniques for removing cataracts include expression of the lens nucleus or aspiration of it through an ultrasonic needle (phacoemulsification). Although there are arguments for and against each technique, the skill and judgment of the surgeon are more important than the method used. Cataract surgery is performed on an outpatient basis and causes very little disability. Modern "extracapsular" cataract surgery leaves the posterior capsule of the lens in the eye; it may become cloudy over time, in which case an opening is easily made with the YAG laser. Despite popular myth, *primary* cataract removal is a surgical procedure and cannot be performed with lasers.

Macular Degeneration

One of the most significant and frustrating causes of visual disability in the older population is age-related macular degeneration. The term is broad and encompasses both mild degrees of atrophy and severe hemorrhagic disease. The cardinal symptom is blurred or distorted central vision, which may develop very gradually in the atrophic forms, or rather suddenly when subretinal vessels bleed or exude fluid. Prompt evaluation is critical since new vessels can grow quite rapidly, but, if recognized, they can be destroyed with laser photocoagulation. However, when

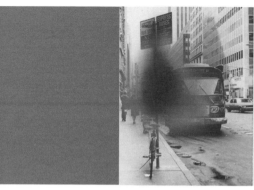

Macular Degeneration
The deterioration of the macula, the central area of the retina, is prevalent among older patients. This illustration shows the area of decreased central vision, called a central scotoma. With macular degeneration, print appears distorted and segments of words may be missing.

they extend beneath the fovea (the center of vision), laser treatment becomes difficult or impossible. Without treatment, the end result of exudative macular degeneration is usually poor, with vision between 20/200 and the ability just to count fingers.

Vision in the atrophic forms of macular degeneration ranges from nearly normal to severely reduced. You may see gross atrophy in the macula, or sometimes the presence of drusen (yellowish spots that represent a degenerative change in the pigment epithelium layer behind the retina). Patients with these findings should be assessed by an ophthalmologist. Note that macular degeneration virtually never extends beyond the macula.

Thus, even though vision may be very poor for reading or working, reassure patients that they will never go totally blind and will always have reasonable side vision that enables them to walk about. Low-vision magnifying devices can be prescribed by doctors who specialize in low-vision rehabilitation so that patients with macular disease may continue to read and do close work.

Laser treatment can help some severe cases, but it does not necessarily prevent recurrence as aging continues. Considerable interest has arisen recently in the potential protective value of antioxidant vitamins and minerals, especially zinc. Experimental

■ Patients with atrophic macular degeneration should be considered for low-vision evaluation. Because the peripheral retina remains relatively normal, magnifying lenses or such devices may provide the patient with a means of continuing to read and perform other near tasks. Selected patients with hemorrhagic macular disease may also benefit from high-magnification lenses or from more powerful low-vision aids, such as a closed-circuit television magnifier.

evidence suggests that oxidative damage and chronic light exposure contribute to retinal aging. However, no firm evidence shows that light or oxidation are actually risk factors in humans, or that any vitamins and minerals have protective value beyond normal dietary amounts. Patients should not become vitamin deficient, and vitamin supplements with zinc may be reasonable; however, large doses are not advisable until a much clearer scientific rationale is established. (The Amsler Grid Eye Test, on page 21, can be used in screening patients for macular degeneration.)

Glaucoma

Glaucoma is often called the "silent thief of sight" because it affects side vision long before central vision is damaged. Thus, sufferers may lose much of their vision before realizing it is gone and seek help too late. For this reason, and because the disease is easily treatable, periodic screening to prevent glaucomatous damage is absolutely vital. Because glaucoma tests are inexpensive and quick, it is unconscionable to omit them from annual geriatric medical exams. For example, pressure testing can be done in any physician's office with the handheld Schiötz tonometer, a small pressure-measuring device that is easy to use and can be handled by technical personnel. A quick look at the optic nerve through an ophthalmoscope will reveal signs of pressure damage (paleness and central excavation or "cupping").

Ordinary open-angle glaucoma affects roughly 2.5 percent of

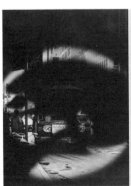

Glaucoma - Chronic elevated eye pressure in susceptible individuals may cause optic nerve atrophy and loss of peripheral vision. Early detection and close medical monitoring can help reduce complications. In advanced glaucoma, print may appear faded and words may be difficult to read.

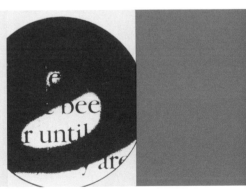

the population over 40, and the incidence rises even higher with age. It is more prevalent in blacks than whites. Glaucoma is defined by elevated pressure within the eye. Although high pressure alone is not proof of progressive glaucoma, intraocular pressures above 22 mm Hg should be considered suspicious until proved otherwise. An ophthalmologic exam will provide such critical techniques as automated visual fields and sophisticated optic nerve evaluation. Pressures over 30 mm Hg are usually treated to minimize the risk of visual loss. Treatment typically involves no more than eyedrops, but if the high pressure persists, excellent surgical procedures are available.

It is important to distinguish chronic *open-angle glaucoma* from *narrow-angle glaucoma*. The latter is a rare acute event in which pressure within the eye rises abruptly with resultant nausea, headache, redness, eye pain, and a rapid loss of vision. Warning signs may be halos around lights (as the cornea becomes hazy) or intermittent soreness of the eyes. Pupillary dilatation may precipitate an attack. *Angle-closure glaucoma* is quite rare, but the risk is highest in the older population. We can identify predisposed eyes by shining a flashlight at the eye from the side, to judge the depth of the chamber between cornea and iris. If the iris is bowed forward so the chamber or "angle" is "shallow," the pupil should not be dilated and the patient should be referred to an ophthalmologist for evaluation. This disease can be prevented in high-risk eyes by making a small hole in the iris with a laser. This procedure prevents the mechanical closure of the angle by opening a passageway for fluid to flow.

Diabetic Retinopathy

Diabetes is a prevalent disease, and most diabetics (both Type I and Type II) will eventually develop retinopathy. Retinopathy cannot be prevented at our present state of knowledge, but many of its visual complications can be prevented if warning signs are recognized early. Early referral of the patient to an ophthalmologist and an interchange of information with the referring physician assures the patient of optimum care.

Diabetic retinopathy falls in two basic categories: *background diabetic retinopathy* (BDR) and *proliferative retinopathy*. BDR involves microaneurysms, hemorrhages, exudates, and the gradual development of retinal edema (which may reduce visual acuity). The pathogenesis involves a dropout of capillaries, which eventually causes enough ischemia to stimulate the growth of new vessels

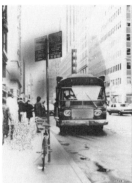

Diabetic Retinopathy - The leaking of retinal blood vessels may occur in advanced or long-term diabetes and affect the macula or the entire retina and vitreous. Not all diabetics develop retinal changes, but the likelihood of retinopathy and cataracts increases with the length of time a person has diabetes.

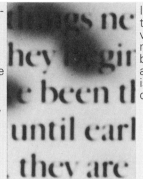

In diabetic retinopathy, reading vision is variable and print may be distorted or blurred. If cataracts are also present, print is hazy as well as distorted.

(called *neovascularization*) that constitute proliferative retinopathy. The problem is that the new vessels in the eye are fragile and bleed easily into the vitreous, which not only blocks vision but leads to scarring that in turn leads to retinal detachment and a potentially blind eye.

Much of the visual loss in BDR can be prevented by selective laser photocoagulation to destroy the areas of microaneurysms and fluid leakage, and to allow the edema to absorb. More extensive photocoagulation in a grid covering the retinal periphery (panretinal photocoagulation) will cause the regression of neovascularization in most cases of proliferative retinopathy. Thus, a large portion of diabetic visual loss is preventable if the retinopathy is recognized early enough on screening exams.

In general, every patient with diabetes should have a dilated fundus exam once a year, and more frequent exams may be advisable after retinopathy has been discovered. The visual symptoms of diabetic retinopathy depend upon the stage. Early BDR may be asymptomatic; macular edema or capillary dropout will cause a gradual dimming of central vision; proliferative disease may cause abrupt or severe visual loss from vitreous hemorrhage. Untreated proliferative disease leads to total blindness.

Corneal Diseases

Corneal diseases are not terribly common, but some are characteristic of older individuals. They often occur as a complication of chronic diseases, such as rheumatoid arthritis and herpes zoster. In general, any thickening or clouding of the cornea will impair vision, often causing glare sensitivity and a loss of contrast perception more than a loss of acuity because of light scattering by the hazy cornea.

Some older individuals are predisposed to edema of the cornea, the risk of which is enhanced by the stress of cataract surgery. Corneal clouding may be an end result of chronic inflammatory disease, such as herpes simplex keratitis. Corneal damage can also occur from a variety of other conditions, including rheumatoid arthritis (peripheral melting of the cornea), dry eyes (severe cases can lead to infections and scarring), herpes zoster (which may affect the cornea somewhat like herpes simplex), and Bell's palsy or other paralytic conditions that leave the cornea exposed (and can result in severe infections or scarring).

In most of these conditions, patients complain of either poor vision or pain. The one exception is an anesthetic cornea from fifth nerve palsy or similar nerve damage. These patients are at a very grave risk of corneal infections and injury because they lack the normal pain-defense mechanism. A brief inspection of the cornea with a flashlight should be a part of every routine physical exam.

Visual Loss from Stroke

The degree of visual loss from a major cerebral stroke depends upon the area of cortical involvement. The most characteristic abnormality is a *homonymous hemianopia*, involving equivalent areas on the same side of the visual field, as a result of

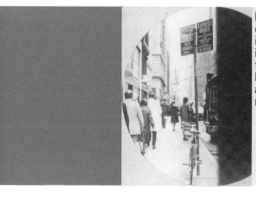

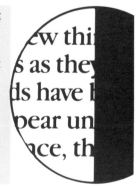

Hemianopia - A defect of the optic pathways in the brain can result in vision loss in half of the visual field. A right homonymous hemianopia can cause reading impairment.

infarction of one cerebral hemisphere. The degree of visual impairment is variable, depending on the site of infarction, and because there is often a degree of macular sparing. Patients may have trouble finding the beginning of lines if the visual loss is to the left or seeing the ends of words if the visual loss is to the right. Patients may consistently bump into objects on one side. Confrontation fields are useful as a simple screening test for hemianopia. Cover one eye, move your fingers or hand in from the four points of the compass while the patient looks directly at the examiner's eye.

Transient visual loss, or amaurosis fugax, is a warning sign of increased risk of stroke or a retinal arterial occlusion (see next section). Attacks may last a few seconds or minutes, and are usually a result of emboli that block a vessel temporarily before breaking up and moving on. Patients with this symptom should be referred for further evaluation.

Vascular
Eye
Conditions

The major vascular problems in older patients, excluding diabetic retinopathy, are arteriosclerosis, hypertension, occlusions of the retinal arteries or veins, and optic nerve ischemia. Arteriosclerosis probably contributes to age-related visual loss in a nonspecific way, as does hypertension.

Acute obstructions of the retinal veins or arteries are not terribly common, but are disastrous visually, since there is an abrupt loss of vision corresponding to the involved area of the retina. *Arterial occlusions* are more severe and less likely to recover. The observation of embolic material within an artery should raise a strong suspicion of carotid or cardiac embolization. *Retinal vein occlusions* are characterized by dilated vessels and hemorrhages throughout the retina. They are often associated with systemic hypertension, but also have a significant association with glaucoma and diabetes. Vein occlusions damage the capillaries much like diabetes, and can cause both macular edema and neovascularization. After central vein occlusions, new vessels may even grow in the iris and cause a particularly severe kind of glaucoma. It is critical to recognize this risk and prevent neovascular glaucoma with panretinal photocoagulation.

Ischemia of an optic nerve causes an abrupt loss of vision, often affecting either the inferior or superior field of view (altitudinal visual loss). Ischemic optic neuropathy or central retinal artery occlusion may also be a sign of giant-cell arteritis (temporal arteritis).

This entity is recognized by finding an elevated sedimentation rate and by temporal artery biopsy. Diagnosis is absolutely critical since, if untreated, the second eye may soon become involved. Systemic corticosteroids are effective in treating temporal arteritis and may even help some eyes with acute ischemic optic neuropathy from other causes.

Retinal Detachment

Retinal detachment as an isolated event is rare and is predominantly a disease of older individuals. It is also a late complication of cataract surgery. The incidence of detachment rises at least 100-fold (to 1 or 2 percent) after cataract extraction, even when the surgery is uncomplicated. Some detachments occur spontaneously as a part of the aging process, when condensation of the vitreous gel pulls upon the retina and causes traction or holes. This contraction often results in "floaters," which are small shadows visible within the eye, especially against a sky or white background. The development of a few floaters is common and usually signifies nothing worrisome. However, a sudden severe accumulation of floaters, especially associated with flashing lights that all come from one direction, could be a warning sign of an impending retinal detachment.

Early recognition and treatment of retinal detachment is important, since the visual result after detachment surgery is variable, and is highly dependent upon the duration of retinal separation. Detachments involving the macular area should be repaired, if possible, within a day or two of occurrence.

Amsler Grid
Eye Test

The Amsler Grid is a symmetrical pattern of squares with a central dot. Pattern changes noted with each eye signal macular retinopathy or other visual pathway disturbance.

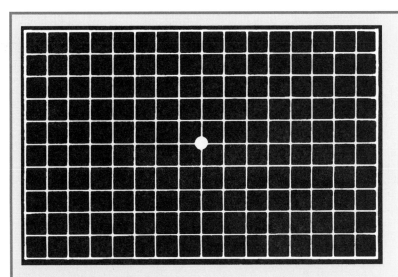

How to Give This Test

1. Patients who usually wear glasses for reading should wear them for this test. The individual should hold the Amsler Grid at the same distance for normal reading material.
2. Instruct the individual to keep both eyes open and to identify the white dot in the center of the grid.
3. Next, the person should close or cover the left eye while continuing to look at the dot.

Ask the individual: Did the squares around the dot change shapes or disappear while covering one eye? Did the lines on the grid appear to be broken, wavy, blurred, or not visible? The patient should repeat this test, covering the right eye.

A "yes" answer for either eye means macular pathology is probably present. However, unless the pupil is dilated for direct observation of the macula, it is risky to draw conclusions from the test. Patients with a positive result on the Amsler Grid should have a complete retinal examination which may include fluorescein angiography and macular visual fields, as well as contrast sensitivity.

Chapter Four

Medication and Vision Impairment
by
Norman Charles, MD

The effects of some systemic medications on vision can be dramatic and irreversible. Because side effects can generally be avoided through the simple strategy of reducing the dosage or substituting an equally effective, but better-tolerated drug, the knowledge of medical specialists must be current in the pharmacology, interactions, and potential side effects of different compounds. This is especially true in today's climate of medical risk management, where popular buzz words are "iatrogenic" and "malpractice."

Document the History

For these reasons, but primarily for the patient's well-being, a careful history taking (and obtaining records from other physicians) with painstaking documentation of prescription drugs (current and over the years) should be routine.

Frank discussion with the patient should always be conducted when you need to weigh the risks and benefits of prescribing a drug that is deemed necessary, but which lists vision loss as a side effect.

Multifactorial Causes of Visual Loss

Although visual loss may be part of a degenerative process, such as glaucoma or macular degeneration, it may be compounded by systemic medications.

Refer to Ophthalmologist for Evaluation

Refer all patients with visual deterioration that may be related to systemic medication to an ophthalmologist.

■ **One caveat:**

Such reference books as the *Physicians' Desk Reference* frequently list "blurred vision" under adverse side effects of drugs. In many cases, this purported side effect involves statistically insignificant or anecdotal reports, sometimes based only on patients' subjective complaints. Included for the sake of completion, these reports of visual disturbance are often not accompanied by clinically demonstrable signs. Many patients in treatment have (or think they have) visual difficulties and are quick to blame the medication for their optical problem. Undoubtedly, some drugs do cause a transient fluctuation in visual clarity without structural pathology in the eye. We have much to learn about such phenomena.

Also be aware that many visual problems can be resolved simply by basic refraction or prescription of low-vision aids.

Drugs Causing Changes in Refraction

Patient Complaint
Diminished reading ability while distance acuity remains satisfactory

Possible cause
Cycloplegia (paralysis of ciliary muscle with loss of accommodation)

Suspect
■ Anticholinergic drugs (tricyclic antidepressants, antianxiety agents, barbiturates, antihistamines, atropine, or scopolamine)

■ Chloroquine and the phenothiazines

Patient management
■ If the drug is necessary to vital function, the patient may continue taking it and, if needed, compensatory reading glasses are prescribed.

■ When taken off the drug, the patient will regain normal accommodative power commensurate with age. *Refer for modification of eyeglass prescription.*

Patient Complaint
Fluctuating visual acuity, sometimes with the expressed fear of "going blind." An alarming and predictable symptom in patients with brittle diabetes or in those undergoing insulin regulation.

Cause
During insulin regulation, the patient has great swings in serum osmolarity. Varying concentrations of glucose enter the human lens capsule, causing daily changes in refraction.

Patient management
■ Reassure the patient that these variations in vision are transient and that a final prescription for eyeglasses will be given when the blood glucose is stabilized. In the interim, the visually disabled patient may require a temporary prescription for glasses.

■ Fluctuating visual acuity may also herald the onset of diabetes mellitus.

Patient Complaint
Myopia (visual blur at distance)

Causative drugs
■ Diuretics and carbonic anhydrase inhibitors may induce transient myopia.

■ Sulfonamides (oral) may also induce transient myopia.

Patient management
■ Change eyeglass prescription.
■ Withdraw the drug. Condition will resolve within several days to a few weeks.

■ Drugs Causing Change in Depth of Focus
Various agents dilate or constrict the pupil, giving rise to a range of complaints.

Key words:
—Mydriasis (pupillary dilation)   —Miosis (pupillary constriction)

In *mydriasis,* where the pupil dilates beyond the normal range and more light is allowed to enter the eye, photophobia (abnormal intolerance to light) may be an accompanying symptom. Some blurring occurs, due to glare. Tinted spectacles may be helpful.

In marked *miosis*, the constricted pupil may cause blurring. Also, the patient will complain that the world appears to be darker than usual. Even moderate miosis in a patient with pre-existing cataracts on the optic axis may precipitate visual disability. An ophthalmologist may elect to treat with mydriatic drops.

■ **Dilated or constricted pupil?**
First, rule out substance abuse.

Miotics may actually have an ameliorating effect on refractive errors by converting the eye to a kind of pinhole camera. Patients often are delighted to discontinue using their eyeglasses and should be encouraged to do so.

■ **Mydriatic drugs**
—Central nervous system stimulants (amphetamines, methylphenidate, cocaine)
—Antihistamines: mild effect on pupil size as well as accommodation
—Anticholinergics, earlier described as cycloplegics, enlarge the pupil. Primary effect: accommodation

■ **Miotic drugs**
—Morphine
—Pilocarpine
—Codeine
—Heroin
—Anticholinesterases

**Drugs Affecting
the Retina
and
Optic Nerve**

Antimalarials (chloroquine, hydroxychloroquine)
The loss of central vision from prolonged administration of antimalarials is well known.

Classic finding

Macular pigmentation in a bull's-eye pattern associated with a central scotoma is related to dose of medication and duration of administration. If detected early, the pathology can be reversed, either totally or partially, by discontinuing the drug.

Is malarial prophylaxis safe?

The answer is yes. Short courses of treatment prescribed for patients traveling to endemic areas do not cause clinical problems.

Long-term use for actual malaria or chronic rheumatoid diseases (lupus erythematosus, discoid lupus) requires ophthalmic monitoring of central visual fields and acuity. With usage of safer dose levels, the incidence of toxic retinopathy due to antimalarials has diminished.

Thioridazine. Used in chronic treatment of psychotic and hyperactive states, it may produce a pigmentary retinopathy and central scotoma. Like chloroquine, side effects are dose- and time-related. If possible, select a safer drug.

Ethambutol. Patients being treated for tuberculosis and related infections are at risk for developing optic neuropathy. *The ophthalmologist should monitor visual acuity, Amsler Grid central field, and color vision every 3 months.*

Chloramphenicol. Chronic use for cystic fibrosis. Toxic effect on optic nerve.

Uncommon or Questionable Retinotoxic Agents

Tamoxifen-related retinopathy has been occasionally reported during treatment of breast carcinoma.

Indomethacin's association with retinopathy has been challenged by retinal specialists who feel that age-related macular degeneration was the cause.

Chlorpromazine has rarely been related to retinopathy.

It should be emphasized that while the retinotoxic potentials of these drugs are less than those of antimalarials and thioridazine, early diagnosis of the occasional case will salvage vision.

Drugs Affecting the Human Lens (Cataractogenic Drugs)

▨ *Corticosteroids*
Topical/Systemic

Caution

—Cause or worsen cataracts

—Cause or worsen glaucoma (especially patients with genetic predisposition or family history)

—May cause side effects that are dosage- and duration-related. Onset may range from days to months.

—*Reversibility*: While discontinuance usually means drop in intraocular pressure or cessation of cataract progression, there are unfortunate exceptions.

■ **Caution**

Corticosteroid-containing eyedrops. Warn patients of hazard of self-medicating on chronic basis. For allergic conjunctivitis, recommend artificial tears, naphazoline, sodium cromolyn, and ice-cold compresses.

Discussion

When indicated, a short-term prescription of corticosteroids, given systemically for 1 week or 2 weeks, rarely produces problems. Topical steroid creams and ointments applied to the skin, including the outer surface of the eyelids, pose little real danger to the globe. *Hazard: Systemic steroids and steroids applied directly to the globe may promote ocular herpes simplex and other opportunistic infections.* Patients requiring long-term steroid therapy should be followed up by an ophthalmologist.

▨ *Psoralens.* PUVA therapy for severe psoriasis requires exposing patients to ultraviolet light. To protect from theoretically possible cataract formation, patients must wear UV-filtering goggles for 24 hours after each treatment. To date, properly conducted PUVA therapy appears to pose no threat to vision.

▓ *Lovastatin.* Indication: hypercholesterolemia. Despite initial reports of worsening of cataracts in some patients and amelioration in others, no reports in the ophthalmic literature have proved that HMG-CoA reductase inhibitors are hazardous to the eye.

Drugs Decreasing Tear Secretion

- ▓ Antihistamines
- ▓ Isotretinoin
- ▓ Anticholinergics
- ▓ Antiparkinsonian agents
- ▓ Beta-adrenergic blocking agents
- ▓ Phenothiazines
- ▓ Tricyclic antidepressants
- ▓ Monoamine oxidase inhibitors

Clinical symptoms are rarely disabling. Rx: over-the-counter artificial tears and lubricant ointments.

Caution
Rule out dry-eye syndrome with blurring of vision due to incomplete corneal wetting in addition to the effect of these drugs on other parts of the eye. Also, a pre-existing dry eye may be made intolerable by these agents.

Suggested Reading

Fraunfelder FT. *Drug-induced Ocular Side Effects and Drug Interactions.* Philadelphia: Lea & Febiger, 1982.

Fraunfelder FT, Meyer SM. The national registry of drug-induced ocular side effects. *J Toxicol Cutan Ocul Toxicol* 1982;1:65-70.

Grant WM. *Toxicology of the Eye,* 2nd ed. Springfield, IL: Charles C. Thomas, 1974.

Koneru PB, Lien EJ, et al. Oculotoxicities of systemically administered drugs. *J Ocul Pharmacol* 1986;2:385-404.

Physicians' Desk Reference, 46th ed. Oradell, NJ: Medical Economics Company, 1992.

Polak BCP. Side effects of drugs and tear secretion. *Ophthalmology* 1987;67:115-117.

Chapter Five

Psychosocial Aspects
of Aging
and
Vision Loss
by
Ann Burack-Weiss, DSW

An understanding of the psychosocial effects of vision loss on the older person is essential to the provision of quality medical care. This understanding promotes patient motivation and compliance with care plans in seemingly intractable situations. The physician's approach to the treatment of the older patient should take into account 1) the interactive effects of vision loss and other losses, 2) adaptive and maladaptive responses to vision loss, and 3) the older person's support system.

Interactive Effects

It is rare to find an elderly person whose only complaint is vision loss. Late life is a time of many losses: health, independence, significant others, and activities that give life meaning. Vision loss interacts with other losses of aging to produce a strain on day-to-day functioning and quality of life.

Physical Losses

The impact of vision loss on an older person with multiple illnesses may be overwhelming. It is not unusual to hear a visually impaired older person say something such as, "I could handle the pain of arthritis. I even got to the point that I could inject the insulin for diabetes. But now that my sight is fading, I don't know how I can go on."

What are some of the effects of medical problems on daily life and the elder's self-image? A decrease in mobility, whatever its physical cause, may precipitate social withdrawal and isolation. Cognitive changes, similarly, result in a shrinking of the elder's world as does hearing loss. Moreover, hearing loss may lead to serious misunderstandings with others, even paranoid ideation. (Although the popular myth of individuals with poor vision having more acute hearing is not true, elders do report that they "see better" when they can hear and "hear better" when they can see. People have been known to lip read instinctively.)

Vision loss has a symbolic significance to the elder. Associated with being "blind," it may represent inclusion in a pitied and stigmatized population. It may awaken a sense of dread. (Blindness is one of the most feared illnesses of Americans, ranking fourth after AIDS, cancer, and Alzheimer's disease.) Vision loss also may signal a lack of privacy as financial and personal papers are read by others.

It is always important to know how the individual elder perceives vision loss and other physical losses. The meanings ascribed will vary. Losses of cognitive, sensory, and motility abilities usually contribute to a sense of vulnerability, dependence on others, and fear of additional loss.

Some elders feel helpless and hopeless. Other elders expect that medical interventions will yield a magical cure. These attitudes may act against compliance with physician care plans.

Social Losses

Retirement and widowhood are common life events that precipitate social consequences. Retirement may involve losses of income, outlets for energy and ideas, socialization opportunities, and status. Widowhood is more than the death of a crucial person — as devastating as that might be. For many women, it also marks a diminution of social standing, activities, friendships, and a cessation of opportunities for sexual expression. Men are more likely to remarry. For those who do not, the primary difference between widows and widowers is that men of the aging cohort are often unaccustomed to the performance of basic household chores; poor nutrition and self-care may result. Elders also experience separations as peers relocate, become homebound, or less communicative.

Physical and social losses interact to diminish the older person's adaptive capacity. However, the older individual will usually respond with coping strategies developed over a lifetime.

Identifying Adaptive and Maladaptive Responses

Elderly people can be expected to express normal emotions of anger, frustration, or sadness over vision impairment as they do over other losses. In fact, those who are the most vocal about the difficulties posed by their impairment often cope best.

Adaptive responses are those in which the elderly person solves problems and uses external resources to achieve optimum adjustment. Maladaptive responses are those in which the older person has become dependent or inactive to an extent that cannot be explained by vision impairment or other health problems. This is sometimes termed "excess disability."

Activities of daily living and social behavior reflect adaptation. Such activities include bathing, dressing, toileting, grooming, preparing meals, feeding, housekeeping, taking medication, managing money, walking outside, riding in a bus, doing the laundry, grocery shopping. For each of these activities (or a selected few), the physician might ask the older patient if he continues to do them alone, has accepted help with them, or has ceased to do them. What are the reasons for giving up an activity? Are the reasons appropriate? For example, the elder with moderate visual impairment who has hypertension can be expected to dress himself. After a stroke, the elder with visual impairment may require help dressing.

Maladaptive responses include a preponderance of activities that the patient has given up since vision loss. At the same time, those activities (often of a social or recreational nature), could indeed be resumed with the help of a family member, home health aide, or rehabilitative training.

Such activities include volunteer work, attendance at a senior center or club; attendance at church or synagogue; participation in sports, cards, or other games; working on a hobby; eating out at restaurants; receiving or visiting friends; taking vacations; or driving.

Further questioning by the physician can distinguish between those patients who continued activities and made adjustments where necessary (using low-vision aids or accepting a ride from a friend), and those who did not continue activities, have not considered alternatives, or rejected those offered out-of-hand.

Older people with visual impairment who present a case of "excess disability" can be helped to do more for themselves. This is not done through the precipitous withdrawal of help, but rather by helping them identify within themselves and their support network remaining strengths, as well as providing opportunities for exercising more control over more aspects of their lives. Many elders with visual impairment can attain such psychosocial goals as enhanced self-esteem, more independent performance of activities of daily living, and maintenance of or increased participation in social and recreational activities if provided an opportunity to discuss their concerns with a caring professional and/or peers.

Elders who feel helpless or hopeless about their abilities may need more than encouragement from the physician. Although antidepressant medication and/or referral to a psychiatrist might be necessary interventions, they are by no means the only ones. There are social agencies in every community with trained staff who are familiar with late-life problems and are available to help older people and their families to explore alternative methods of care and continuation of activities.

The Support System

Over three decades of research has confirmed that most families do not "dump" their elderly into nursing homes or otherwise depend upon formal agencies or governmental assistance. Over 80 percent of care to the elderly is provided by family; outside help is sought only when the financial and emotional resources of the family are exhausted. Institutional care is used mostly by the very old, those with no families, and those with cognitive impairments.

Most often, the primary caregiver is a middle-aged daughter struggling to reconcile her own needs or the needs of a husband and children with those of an aged parent, creating "a sandwich generation" with demands on both sides. More women are now entering the present workforce than in previous generations and more of these women are feeling entitled to time for themselves.

Yet another common pattern in caregiving is the significant amount of spousal care, usually by wives of disabled husbands. Late-life marriage is often characterized by the mutual dependence of a couple who are impaired in different ways. While such an alliance is touching to onlookers, it is also exceedingly fragile: The slightest change in physical functioning of either partner places both in jeopardy.

Neighbors and friends often play a role in providing social support to the elderly. Although they may not assume major responsibility for decision making or daily care, they can provide emotional support as well as help in shopping, errands, and a sense of security simply by their presence close at hand.

The elder with visual impairment will rely heavily on an "informal" support system for care — often unaware of availability of "formal" services provided by social and health-care agencies. A physician's referral to such sources of support can be very beneficial.

■ Case Study

At the other extreme is the older person who may receive too much care, such as Mrs. G, an 84-year-old woman, who lives alone. She worked as a secretary until her retirement, and for 10 years after retirement was a volunteer in the Foster Grandparent Program. She left that work when her husband had a stroke, and cared for him at home until his death three years later. Although her medical situation is fairly stable, two years ago she was diagnosed as having macular degeneration and, since that time, has grown increasingly homebound and frail.

She has two children: a son who lives out of state and a daughter who lives nearby. They persuaded her to accept a live-in home attendant a year ago. At her last medical appointment, she expressed a sense of hopelessness: "There is nothing left for me to live for." She praised the home attendant and was proud of her children for providing so well for her, but found time hanging heavily on her hands, as she can no longer read and has no household tasks to occupy her time.

The primary care physician identified hers as a case of "excess disability," contributing to hopelessness and helplessness. Knowing Mrs. G's past history, he was able to put her in touch with still-existing personal strengths. He encouraged her toward rehabilitative efforts and assuming responsibility for the tasks in her home she could still perform. He referred her to a low-vision clinic where she received a magnifying lens to assist in reading. He reassured her adult children that she could perform more independently. He also referred her to a community agency specializing in services to the aged visually impaired where she could participate in a peer-support group.

The Physician's Role in Intervention

Older people with visual impairment may lose confidence in themselves and their abilities to manage their daily lives. Their fear and anxiety are often reinforced by overprotective family members. The opinion of the elder's physician is usually sought and respected by elders and families, particularly as it relates to the degree of acceptable risk in a living situation.

A typical scenario is the adult child who insists on a homecare attendant while the incapacitated parent steadfastly insists that he can live alone. The physician's reinforcement of the need for care can be helpful and supportive at this point.

Chapter Six

Practice Management: The Office Environment
by
Clare M. Hood, RN, MA

For some older persons, forays into the outside world might be diminishing, and a visit to the doctor in an office setting becomes a significant event. The visit is planned well in advance, schedules checked, and every effort made to be on time, if not early. The visit is frequently viewed with anxiety, for fear that symptoms cannot be treated or cured and that could result in a reduction of the quality of life and one step closer to dependency. Other patients might fear having to take medications and worry about the cost. Therefore, the physician and staff should work together to create an environment and an atmosphere in which the older patient feels welcome, as secure as possible, and, above all, is given time to discuss problems with both the doctor and the staff, time to review directions, and to repeat them back.

The following suggestions are helpful in interacting with any older person, but in particular the patient with low vision who may also have a hearing loss.

Environmental Considerations in the Medical Facility

Medical facilities vary in layout and design. Whether high-tech or "old-fashioned," most offices contain some environmental features that are difficult for any older person with vision loss. These features may affect the perceived delivery of health care. Let's walk through a visit through the eyes of a patient, starting with initial access to the physician's office.

Entrance. Is there parking? Does the approach to the office require climbing stairs and is there an elevator? Can the patient find the right office entrance? Is there a bell to be rung?

Stairs. Unless a definite contrast is evident between the edge of the drop-off and the first step, the individual may not see the stairs. Easy solutions include a well-lighted entryway and stairs marked with a light or with a contrasting strip of tape at the top and bottom steps. Ideally, bannisters should extend the full length of the stairway.

Elevator. Are the buttons marked in large print and is each floor identified with large numbers on the walls opposite the elevator door so the person can identify the floor? Is there a railing in the elevator for the person to hold on to?

Reception area. The receptionist should be visible from the door, if possible. In this way, the patient can receive clear directions immediately upon entering and assistance, if necessary. The receptionist should greet the patient by name and direct the person to approach the reception desk. The receptionist should then give explicit directions to the waiting room, the bathroom, the coat rack, and other areas the patient may need.

Waiting room. Organize the waiting room and office in clearly delineated spaces, with contrasting furniture, walls, and rugs. Keep passageways uncluttered.

Low magazine tables in the center of the room invite trouble. Place them between chairs and use lighting that shines on reading material, but not in the patient's face. Provide large-print books, newspapers, pamphlets, and fliers about visual and other medical problems.

Set aside quiet, private space for staff interaction with the patient. Make sure there is adequate lighting at the receptionist's and billing workspaces.

Color contrast for clearer visibility. Consider painting the waiting room and examining rooms with nongloss paint in contrasting colors, especially in the hallways, on the doors, and baseboards. The strategy of painting the baseboard with a contrasting, or darker, color distinguishes the edge of the wall from the floor. Carpeting should be a solid color. Avoid complex patterns. Avoid wallpaper with strong vertical lines; to a patient with an eye disease, these lines may look wavy. Chairs and tables should stand out against a solid background. Chairs should be at a comfortable height, with arms that the patient can use for support and, preferably, in a material that can be easily washed. The legs of the chairs should be straight to minimize tripping.

Restrooms. The doors should be large enough to accommodate a wheelchair or a walker, and the toilet stalls should have railings. Symbols or signs in large print are helpful for identification of the restroom itself. Use contrasting colors for the toilet stall, sink, and paper dispenser. The sinks should have large, easily maneuvered faucets. Mark the hot-water faucet with a large red dot on the tap. Make sure that the paper-cup dispenser in the bathroom is easily located.

Helping Patients with Dual-Sensory Loss

Patients with both vision and hearing loss need a special approach. Therefore, it is important that the physician and staff indicate this situation on the patient's card or record so that special directions can be given early in the patient's contact with the office.

Minimize background noise, including music. Instead of a soothing effect, music can create special difficulties for the person with a hearing loss. Loud conversation, ringing telephones, and computer hums could contribute to the background noise that may be annoying and confusing to the patient with hearing impairment. To avoid surprise, speak before touching the person. Speak directly to the person and introduce other staff members who are present.

Techniques

Speak more clearly and slowly than usual and at close range. Don't shout.

Modulate your voice so that you do not shout. Shouting often sounds as if you are angry or very upset. Invest in a portable amplifier to communicate with the patient with a hearing loss who is not wearing a hearing aid. Confirm appointments in writing to assist the patient who may not be able to take the information over the telephone or may not have heard it clearly.

If communication is difficult, speak to a family member, a friend, or a caregiver, and ask what communication methods work

Sighted Guide Technique

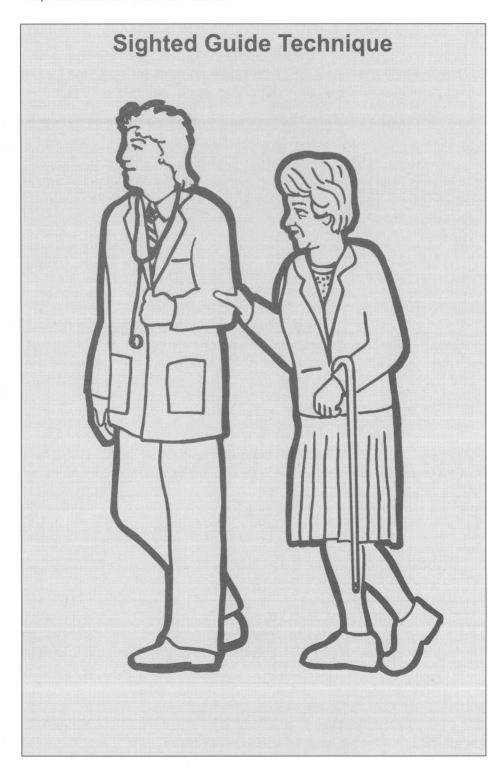

■ Sighted Guide Technique

A special technique originally developed for blind people can be equally useful for guiding individuals who are unsure of their bearings. The person can feel and follow the guide's direction while navigating in an unfamiliar office.

Not all older people require assistance, and many cherish their independence. Therefore, ask patients with low vision if they need help getting into the various parts of the office. Anticipating need prevents embarrassment

The person with low vision is instructed to hold the guide's arm lightly above the elbow and to allow the guide to walk one-half step ahead. Although this method allows the individual to feel the direction, warnings still need to be given about steps, ramps, and narrow corridors.

■ Directions

Going through narrow door or passage. The guide presses the guiding arm backward so that the person moves back in single file far enough to prevent stepping on the guide's heels.

Stairs. Again, the individual walks one stair step behind, holding the guide's upper arm with one hand and the handrail with the other.

Approaching a chair. Guide the person's arm to the back or side arm of the chair, allowing the person to determine where to sit.

■ Sighted Guide Technique for Person Requiring Extra Support

The guide should bend the supporting arm parallel to the ground so that the patient can apply weight to the guide's arm, thus securing additional support.

■ Remember:

Orientation to the environment can be affected by the medications or combination of medications that the older individual is taking. If problems with ambulating or balance result, consider changing the time or medications or changing the medications themselves. Consider the use of a support cane, four-prong cane, or walkers on wheels.

best for that patient. This is particularly important with patients who have difficulty speaking due to neurological conditions, or who do not understand or speak English.

Avoid using only hand or head movements to indicate direction. The patient with reduced vision may not be able to see these gestures and will perceive you as not having communicated at all.

Scheduling Appointments

For a patient with vision impairment, early morning appointments and traveling when it's dark are difficult. Confirm appointments to be sure that the person has the correct date and time. Write appointment dates in large letters, using black ink.

Billing

Some patients may request to have the bill read to them. Have a signature guide available for patients to sign their names on the forms or their checks.

Ambulation Consideration in the Medical Office

Notice how the patient gets around the office. Does the person need the help of another individual? Is the patient using a cane or walker? Should the patient be using a cane or walker? Is the patient unsure or unsteady?

Preparation for the Examination

Make certain that the dressing room is well lighted and that there is a sturdy chair. Older adults with vision loss may need help identifying the front and back of the gown and the location of the clothes hooks on the wall.

Examination Procedures

Tell the patient what procedure to anticipate and identify each procedure before starting. Face the patient when giving directions or describing a procedure.

Patient Education

Print directions for the patient in large print with a black felt-tipped pen. In this way, patients may review directions and instructions when they get home.

Summary

With a little thought and strategic planning, modifications can easily be incorporated into your preexisting office setting and routine, which can contribute to the patient's positive experience. A patient who feels comfortable and who has established communication with the physician and the staff is a person who will make every effort to follow directions and will direct energy to getting well and maintaining good health.

References

Lighthouse Consumer Catalog. New York: Lighthouse Consumer Products, 1991.

Lighthouse Low Vision Catalog, 7th ed. New York: Lighthouse Low Vision Products, 1992.

Self-Help/Mutual Aid Support Groups for Visually Impaired Older People: A Guide and Directory. New York: Lighthouse National Center for Vision and Aging, The Lighthouse Inc., 1990.

Sound and Sight: Your Second Fifty Years. New York: Lighthouse National Center for Vision and Aging, The Lighthouse Inc., 1990.

Faye EE (ed). *Clinical Low Vision,* 2nd ed. Boston: Little, Brown and Company, 1984, chap 13.

Genensky S, Berry S, Bikson TH, Bikson TK. *Visual Environmental Adaptive Problems of the Partially Sighted.* Santa Monica, CA: Center for the Partially Sighted, 1979 (CPS-100-HEW).

Karp A. *Hearing impairment.* In Faye EE (ed). *Clinical Low Vision,* 2nd ed. Boston: Little, Brown and Company, 1984, pp 395-413.

Pamphlets on Eye Disease and Vision

American Academy of Ophthalmology
P.O. Box 7424
San Francisco, CA 94120-7424

American Optometric Association
243 N. Lindbergh Blvd.
St. Louis, MO 63141

Chapter Seven

Staff Instruction and Training
by
Karen R. Seidman, MPA

The messages that members of the staff convey to patients, verbally and nonverbally, contribute to the patient's overall comfort level and response to the practice. For this reason, it is important for all staff members — clerical, administrative, and professional — to support by their actions the practice's commitment to provide for the special needs of patients with age-related vision problems.

Many offices have staff training programs and regularly scheduled meetings for education and discussion of various topics and issues. At these meetings, staff members can learn to recognize the most common problems associated with vision loss and to understand when and how to intervene to assist the patient.

Staff Instruction

A staff meeting directed to sensitizing staff members to the needs of visually impaired patients as they go through the regular office routine should seek to:

- *Instruct in basic, practical language* about the most prevalent forms of vision loss in the elderly and the impact on a person's ability to function.

- *Dispel misconceptions* about the capabilities of the older, visually impaired patient.

- *Encourage staff at all levels to identify activities* in their usual interaction with patients, which might be more difficult when the patient has a vision problem. (A good example is the process of filling out forms.)

- *Stimulate discussion of practical solutions* to problems the patients with low vision in the practice may encounter during the office visit.

■ *Explain to staff any environmental modifications* already made or planned to emphasize the team commitment to making the office more "low-vision patient friendly."

Common Problems and Interventions

Identification

The new patient. Upon first encounter, it may not be immediately apparent that the person is visually or hearing impaired. The patient may not think that the problem is relevant to the office visit, may be reluctant to mention it, or be unaware of the severity of the problem. The receptionist and other staff members should observe the patient moving about the waiting room and office and take note of the patient's responsiveness to questions and the ability to fill out forms.

Particular difficulties should be charted in such a way that any staff member who interacts with the patient will be alerted to the patient's needs. By watching the patient's body language and method of communication during the initial contact and by flagging certain signs and symptoms for the physician to see, staff can actively contribute to the diagnostic and management process.

The return patient. When the patient is known to have a vision problem, color coding or flagging the section of the patient's chart visible to the staff will signal that the patient might require help, or an assistive device, to complete certain activities.

> ■ Clue in the appointment secretary to fill out an appointment card so that the patient can read it without help by writing "large print/dark pen" or other instructions on a flagged chart.

Forms

The forms associated with medical office visits (medical history, insurance, informed consents, etc.) can present three problems to the person with low vision:

1. Reading them;
2. Filling them out; and
3. Signing them.

> ■ **Forms that work**
>
> Forms the patient must read or sign should be designed with easily readable print and with good contrast between ink and paper colors. Try to avoid preprinted forms that are pale in tone. Use the office copier to enlarge and darken print on forms and office correspondence to patients. Allow patients to take home more readable copies of any instructions, waivers, releases, etc.
>
> Look critically at the workstations in the office where patients are usually handed forms. Analyze the conditions under which patients must read or fill them out. Equipping these workstations with a few assistive devices (i.e., lighting, bold-line pens) may enable patients to complete these tasks on their own.

Signing Forms

Signing consents, claim forms, releases, checks, etc., can be a daunting task to the patient with vision loss. Here are some suggestions:

- *Signature on file.* To minimize the number of insurance forms to be signed, the patient can sign a "signature on file" statement, which only needs to be signed once to authorize insurance billing.

- *An ink stamp* with the name of the physician or group practice reduces the amount of writing required to fill out a check.

- *Help in signing names.* Older patients with age-related vision loss often express self-consciousness about their inability to sign their names clearly or to keep their signature on a straight line. Some solutions are:

  —*Use a black, felt-tipped pen* to darken the line on which the patient must sign.

  —*Use a signature guide* (a black, plastic 3" x 5" card with a rectangular cutout) that can be made or purchased and placed over the signature block on the form or the check to guide the patient's signature.

  —*Give explicit instructions* or help position the patient's pen on the signature line.

Good Lighting

Good lighting may be important to improve a patient's ability to read print. In addition to regular overhead lighting, a lamp with a movable arm is particularly helpful at a workstation because it can be positioned to maximum advantage for each patient's needs. Staff at the workstation should be instructed in the proper way to adjust the lamp and should routinely ask patients if they need more or less light to read by or to see to sign documents.

Confidentiality

When patients with low vision cannot read required forms for themselves, staff members should be prepared to read the text aloud to them. However, staff should be aware of the need to preserve the patient's confidentiality. This is especially critical when reading sensitive material aloud to the patient and when the workstation is near other patients. Wherever possible, private space should be provided. Informed consents, releases, and other forms should be modified to include a statement for the patient to sign, stating that the information has been read and that he or she has understood it.

Getting Around the Office

Some older patients with vision loss, especially those new to the practice, may have difficulty finding their way around the office.

- *Use clear, descriptive instructions* to explain how to get to the restroom, changing room, or examination room.

- *Be specific.* Use color codes, numbers, and landmarks in your directions. Say, "The examination room is the third door on the right with the large number 1 on it."

- *Staff should act as a sighted guide for patients* who are hesitant to manage on their own or are unable to do so.

As a final note, the attitude of every staff member is a significant factor in building patient satisfaction and follow-up office visits. When in-service training prepares staff members to understand the potential difficulties that older patients with visual impairment may have, they can anticipate the problem areas of the office routine and can incorporate strategies to help those patients get the most from their interactions with the practice.

Chapter Eight

Evaluating
the Living
Situation
by
Clare M. Hood, RN, MA
and
Eleanor E. Faye, MD, FACS

Is the living environment of the elderly patient with low vision as hazard-free as possible or is it an obstacle course, fraught with dark stairwells, shredded carpets, a tangle of electric-light cords, three-legged footstools, and an occasional sleeping cat? How supportive is the support system? Is the home front a battle zone or a comfort area? This type of information is usually not a primary consideration during an initial office visit. The importance of the quality of the home environment is more apparent after the medical evaluation of the patient when the patient's abilities and limitations have been established and plans for continuing care are formulated.

Although a patient generally has some idea of personal limitations, family members and other household companions of the person with reduced vision often do not have an understanding of just what the person is able or unable to do. They are not sure when to help or in what areas. There is uncertainty about how the eye condition affects functional ability and how to guide the person in modifying the home environment, daily living tasks, or leisure activities.

In order to assess the living situation, we recommend that the primary care physician or another health-care professional visit the home, if at all possible. The health-care professional or vision rehabilitation specialist can determine the division of labor in a household, and instruct the key person in the desired regimen to ensure that the patient does not neglect any aspect of care. Involving the caregivers (family, friends, and home health-care personnel) and patient in a practical management plan can build on the strengths of the patient. Every attempt can be made to modify tasks and environment so that the patient is able to retain independence, even on a somewhat limited level.

Questions, observations, and discussion should include the following categories:

- Eye and medical information
- Environmental adaptations for daily living
- Safety and security hints
- Magnification
- Optical and nonoptical devices
- Lighting
- Color and vision
- Community resources

■ Eye and Medical Information

— How does the patient's eye disorder affect ability to function, especially in the ability to get about, to read, and to perform daily activities, such as seeing food on the plate, shopping, and dressing?

— Does the patient use optical devices or need instruction in their use?

— Does the eye condition suggest specific lighting requirements or need for color contrast in the work or living areas?

— What is the effect of the person's medical condition on function in general (for example, in diabetes or cardiovascular disease)?

— Are the medications labeled in large print as to dosage, time of day to be taken, and other precautions or directions?

— Side effects of medications should be reviewed and expiration dates checked on eyedrops or any over-the-counter products.

— If a person is visually impaired, a hearing assessment is indicated to minimize the possibility that the person has a dual sensory loss.

Environmental
Adaptations
for
Daily Living

Household activities. It is important to develop a realistic picture of the patient's ability to participate in activities of daily living, including shopping, cooking, and self-care. A well-motivated person with some support should be able to carry out, with modifications, a nutritional and medical regimen, and continue valued hobbies and recreational activities.

Household organization. During assessment of the living situation, it is important to determine the following:

- Does the patient live alone or with others?

- On whom does the patient rely for help?

- How do the housemates feel about the patient's capacity for independence?

- What is the division of labor within the household?

- What activities can the patient carry out safely?

Obstacles

With a few strategic modifications, most living quarters can be converted into a safer place: Remove obstacles, provide optical magnification or large-print materials, use color contrast, tactile markers, and lighting.

- Always shut doors; do not leave them half-open.

- Put chairs back in place; whenever possible position them against walls.

- Clear all overhead obstructions, such as kitchen or bathroom cabinets and doors.

- Remove small objects on the floor, such as footstools.

- Keep hallways uncluttered.

Indeed, almost any object can be experienced as an obstacle if the person cannot see it. If objects have a set place, their location can be anticipated by the person with visual impairment.

Depending upon the particular vision impairment, the visual field may be obstructed in a variety of ways. For example, in macular degeneration, objects in the area of central vision may be obscured. In glaucoma, peripheral vision may be diminished; therefore, be aware of potential obstacles in either visual field.

Safety
and
Security Hints

- List emergency telephone numbers in large, bold print near the telephone or program them into an electronic telephone.

- Review safety techniques in bathroom, kitchen, hallways.

- Identify exits.

- Mark stove, oven, and microwave dials.

- Replace batteries on regular schedule in smoke detector.

- Make sure locks can be manipulated, and keys are identified either with contrasting colors or large labels. Put a light over or near the door.

- Make sure doorbell and telephone can be heard.

- If appropriate, notify the fire and police departments of the patient's needs.

Magnification

The person with visual impairment often needs advice in simple techniques of magnification, such as moving closer to the television screen, or using the prescribed magnifying glasses, hand magnifiers, or stand magnifiers (optical aids). Nonoptical devices supplement optical aids to assist in reading and writing.

Optical devices

Optical aids should be prescribed by a low-vision specialist to ensure that the special needs of the individual are accommodated. These devices enhance both distance and reading sight. Some examples:

- High-power reading lenses

- Hand-held or stand (page-mounted) magnifiers

- Telescopes for distance and near vision, including spectacle-mounted telescopes

- Tinted lenses

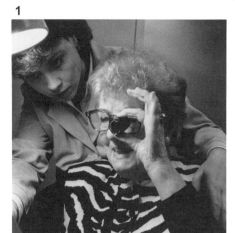

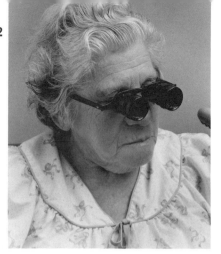

Low-Vision Devices

1. **Hand-held monocular telescope for spotting distant objects**

2. **Spectacle telescope for viewing TV**

3. **Prism glasses for near-work**

4. **High-powered magnifying lens for reading small print**

5. **Hand-held monocular telescope used for near-vision**

6. **State-of-the-art binocular telescopes for varying focal ranges.**

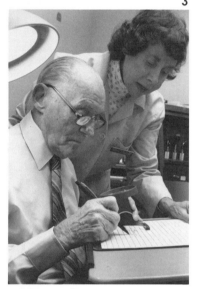

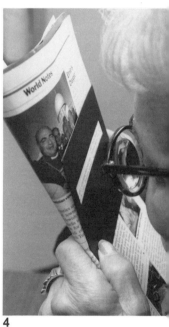

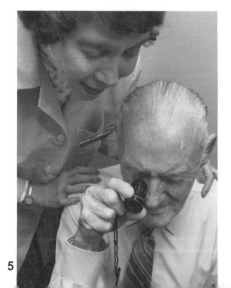

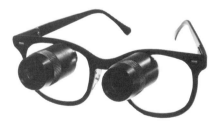

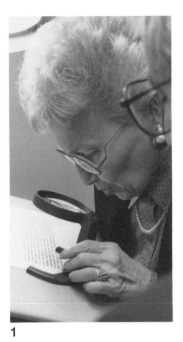

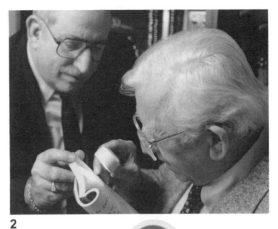

1

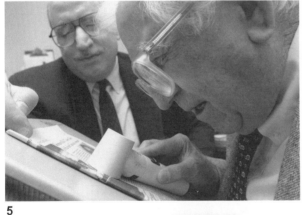

2

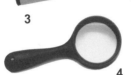

3

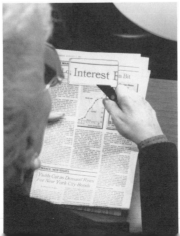

4

5

6

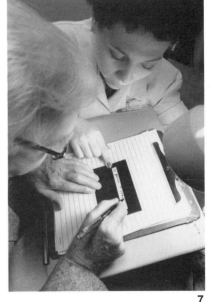

7

Low-Vision Devices

1. Stand magnifier for reading
2. Hand-held magnifier for reading
3. Illuminated stand magnifier
4. Hand magnifier
5. Illuminated magnifier used for reading
6. Rectangular hand magnifier
7. Signature guide and good illumination

Nonoptical and accessory devices

- Felt-tipped pens

- Tactile markers

- Sewing needles with large or hinged eyes and needle threaders

- Talking clocks, watches, and calculators

- Large-numeral telephones, clocks, calculators, timers, and thermostats

- Fluorescent markers

- Flashlights

- Talking books (books on tape)

- Large-print reading materials, games, playing cards

The local public library is a resource for large-print books as well as books on tape, and talking books are available from the Library of Congress.

Large-print materials can make the difference between the elderly person being able to read with ease or haltingly.

High-tech aids

A wide variety of high-tech devices complement optical aids, and allow the low-vision person to read and write with relative ease. Some examples:

- Computer magnification systems, such as the video magnifier (CCTV) that enlarges print material on a television monitor for reading

- Large-print display software to attach to computers

- Portable video (and electronic) magnifiers for reading and writing

- Optical scanners that turn typeset and typewritten material into synthetic speech

Lighting

Good lighting is one of the simplest and least costly ways to manage the environment. Lighting is critical for safety and performance, often making it possible for a low-vision patient to continue reading, eating, sewing, and writing.

Persons over 65 with normal vision need three times more light than persons in their 20s to engage in the same tasks. Illumination for a specific patient depends on that person's vision impairment. What may be adequate lighting for one individual may seem excessive to another. In cataracts, for example, too much light can cause a problem by creating glare.

In an area designated for general use, such as living room or kitchen, it is important to have even illumination, ideally with rheostat controls. Both the type of light used and its placement should be evaluated:

- *Fluorescent lighting.* Provides good overall illumination, but can cause glare if daylight bulbs or cold blue light is used. Energy-saving fluorescent bulbs that are similar to warm incandescent light are available. Halogen light may also cause glare.

- *Spot incandescent lighting.* Use spot lighting wherever possible. Lampshades should be opaque, shielding the light source and at the same time directing the light onto a work area.

- *Direct sources of bright light.* Filter natural sunlight with thin curtains that permit light to pass through. Filter artificial lighting with lampshades.

- *Strategic placement of lights.* Avoid distracting reflections from the TV screen or from windows.

Color and Vision

Often, elderly persons with low vision have imperfect color vision. Use contrasting colors so that objects are clearly seen. For example, dark plates on light place mats, white or light-colored foods on dark plates, darker or bright-colored foods on white plates, water in a red or a blue glass. Also, to avoid accidents, chair coverings should stand out against the carpet color and be easily seen against wall coverings. If contrast is lacking, the person may trip or fall.

■ In the Home

—*Medications.* Since many medications are identified by color, there is potential confusion with "look-alike" pills. Medication should be identified by large-print labels.

—*Objects needing to be easily located.* Household utensils or equipment should be chosen with color contrast in mind or marked with colored tape to create contrast.

—*Work areas.* Table surfaces used as workspace should contrast with the project materials for easy distinction.

—*Meals.* Plates, flatware, tablecloths, and foods should contrast in color and brightness to enhance their visibility. They should be arranged consistently to make finding the food and tableware as simple as possible.

—*Reading.* Some low-vision patients find that placing a transparent yellow sheet over a page of print while reading helps to clarify the image.

—*Tactile markers, felt adhesives, textured tiles, carpet.* Tactile markers have a limited use in the home for patients who cannot use color clues or contrast. Plastic material may be used to form dots that patients can use to identify stove or thermostat dials.

■ Community Resources

—Refer for transport to medical care, senior centers, exercise classes, shopping, social events, and religious centers.
—Provide information and addresses of rehabilitation agencies.
—Encourage and support the family and caregivers in obtaining help.
—Advise on self-help and support groups.
—Give information on adaptive products.

The Lighthouse National Center for Vision and Aging is a major resource that can provide references to local low-vision specialists, community resources, suppliers of adaptive devices, and support groups.

Chapter Nine

Avoiding
Falls
by
Rein Tideiksaar, PhD

Falls are a common health problem for elderly people. Each year, up to 50 percent of persons aged 65 and older at home or in nursing facilities fall. Many suffer multiple falling episodes with serious consequences, such as hip fracture, particularly in the presence of osteoporosis. In the absence of injury, elderly persons can develop a fear of further falls that may lead to a restriction of activities and immobility.

Most falls are associated with ordinary activities, such as walking on uneven ground, climbing or descending steps, transferring on and off chairs, beds, toilets, and reaching up or bending down to retrieve or place objects. Ultimately, falls occur when the activity results in a loss of balance, and the customary neuromuscular systems responsible for compensation fail.

Generally, there are many reasons for older people to be prone to falls. The reasons can be such intrinsic factors as transient and chronic neurologic, musculoskeletal, and cardiovascular disorders that affect vision, gait, balance, muscle strength, and blood pressure. The environmental factors that promote instability are poor lighting, steep steps, slippery or uneven floor surfaces, carpeting, improper footwear, or wrong type of cane.

The risk of falling increases in direct proportion to the number of complicating disorders and environmental hazards. In devising strategies to predict and prevent falls for each patient at risk, or for those who have already fallen, each intrinsic and extrinsic element must be carefully considered.

Vision
and
Falls

Vision plays a critical role in maintaining postural stability or balance. The visual system works in conjunction with the vestibular and proprioceptive systems to help orient the body in space and to stabilize it during ambulation. Good eyesight is necessary for a person to perceive the surrounding environment clearly and to analyze prevailing conditions correctly. Impaired vision leads to slips and trips, loss of balance, and falls.

Age-related vision changes and disease states, as discussed in Chapter 3, affect visual acuity, adaptation to darkness, brightness discrimination, accommodation, glare recovery, depth perception, contrast sensitivity, and peripheral vision.

Although elderly people may not experience severe visual impairment as a result of these changes, the decline in visual function is sufficient to heighten the risk of falling. This is especially true when, in conjunction with a poorly illuminated visual environment, objects in the pathway (e.g., upended rug edges, steps, door thresholds) are difficult to perceive.

While many changes in visual function cannot be reversed, much can be done to overcome their effects by modifying the environment of the elderly person. To ensure proper adaptation of the environment, it is essential first to observe the person moving about and to assess specific visual requirements.

To accomplish this objective, community-residing persons can be referred to a vision rehabilitation agency that provides staff trained to assess the home environment and offer modification suggestions to promote safety and autonomy.

Adapting the Visual Environment

The aspect of the environment most easily adapted to improve vision and reduce fall risk is lighting.

Illumination

Illumination is essential to vision, and elderly people require an increased level of illumination because of the decline in retinal sensitivity that accompanies the aging process. However, the rule of thumb that elderly people require two or three times more light than younger people is a generalization. There are occasional visual conditions in which lower lighting levels may be more appropriate. For instance, persons with cataracts tend to be sensitive to bright lights. Glare may actually impair vision and increase the risk of falling.

Under the best circumstances, the control of lighting levels should rest in the hands of the individual so that each person is able to regulate and maintain a level of lighting that is both visually comfortable and optimal for safe mobility. Some older adults may economize on lighting to control costs of electric bills.

> ■ To enable individuals to control lighting levels, use three-way light bulbs or rheostat light switches or energy-efficient bulbs that can be used in standard fixtures.

Effective Lighting Sources

The quality of lighting is important to consider. Full-spectrum fluorescent lighting is commonly used for overall illumination in stores, public buildings, and kitchens. Although "blue" fluorescent lighting simulates natural sunlight and provides a supply of lighting that is evenly spread, continuous, and free of shadows, some patients with cataracts or corneal problems will complain of increased glare. Most persons prefer the quality of light produced by a bulb in the yellow spectrum, whether fluorescent or incandescent.

Strategic Lighting

Extra lighting may be needed in certain high-risk fall locations, such as the bedroom, stairs, halls, and bathroom. Adequate lighting should be planned for the person who must get up during the night to go to the bathroom. The route may have several fall hazards, such as rug edges, door saddles, and low-lying furniture that is difficult to see. A bedside lamp with a secure base that will not tip over, a bedside light within easy reach that is attached to a headboard, or the addition of nightlights are helpful.

Staircases should have lighting fixtures placed below eye level and near the top and bottom steps. This lighting helps people judge the height of the steps and avoid tripping.

Abrupt
Lighting
Changes

The ability of the eyes to adapt to changes in illumination decreases with age. Remember that any sudden change in lighting intensity can lead to a momentary decrease in customary visual acuity. The use of rheostat light switches that vary the amount of light available ensures an even distribution of light and prevents sudden shifts in illumination that may occur from the use of toggle light switches.

Lighting
Access

All environmental lighting should be readily accessible to everyone, especially to individuals with low vision.

- *Light switches* should be approximately 32 inches from the floor, and located directly on the outside or inside of doorways. This helps to orient the person walking across a darkened room to turn on a light.

- *Light switchplates* should be of a color that contrasts with that of the wall to allow for visibility. If the colors of the wall and switchplate are identical, color contrasting tape around the borders of the switchplate will enhance its visibility.

- A *small light* located within the switch or illuminated switchplates allows for visibility and access at night.

- *Pressure-type light* controls are easier to use than standard toggle switches.

- *Lamps* that turn on by a simple touch are available.

- *Ceiling lights* controlled by a pull cord should have a cord that hangs at eye level, to avoid excessive reaching up and risking a loss of balance.

- *Light timers*, preset for certain times, are helpful if the addition of light switches is not feasible.

Glare May
Cause Falls

Glare from sunlight or any other light source, including unshielded light sources, reflections on polished floors, tabletops, furniture, and television screens may impair vision.

- To eliminate sunlight streaming through windows, use thin draperies or venetian blinds unless they excessively reduce the amount of available light.

- Polarized window glass or tinted mylar shades will eliminate glare without loss of light. Glare from unshielded light sources can be reduced by using frosted light bulbs and placing shades on exposed bulbs.

- To control floor glare from light or sunlight on highly polished, waxed floors, use carpets or nonslip floor finishes that diffuse rather than reflect light.

- Reposition lamps that cause glare.

- Use wall-mounted valances or cove lighting to conceal the source of light and spread it indirectly upon the ceiling and floor to eliminate glare.

- To eliminate furniture surface glare, use matte or dull surfaces on tabletops and nonreflective material on chair seats.

Environmental
Areas and
Objects

In addition to improving lighting conditions, consider other modifications in enhancing visual function.

- Pay attention to floor surfaces. Plain-colored, unpatterned floor coverings are less confusing visually than carpets or tiles with floral or checked patterns that may lead to misjudgment of spatial distances. Door thresholds or saddles may not be seen clearly if they are of a color similar to the surrounding floor. This problem can be eliminated by placing brightly colored nonslip adhesive strips along the length of the threshold or by painting thresholds a contrasting color.

- Utilize contrasting color to attract attention to potentially hazardous elements of the environment. Risers and treads on steps and stairways should not be painted or carpeted the same color, or carpeted with patterned material. Both may hamper recognition of step height and depth. Placing brightly colored orange or yellow nonslip adhesive strips along the length of each step will help with detection.

- Painted or papered stairway walls in a color lighter than the stairs can highlight the steps and enhance illumination as well.

- Objects that serve as balance supports, such as bannisters and toilet and bathtub grab bars, should be visually highlighted by contrasting their color from the background.

Suggested Reading

Baker SP, Harvey AH. Fall injuries in the elderly. *Clin Geriatr Med* 1985;1:501.

Kennedy TE, Coppard LC (eds). The prevention of falls in later life. *Dan Med Bull* 1987;34(suppl 4):1.

Tideiksaar R. *Falling in Old Age: Its Prevention and Treatment.* New York: Springer Publishing Company, 1989.

Chapter Ten

The Outdoors
by
William R. Wiener, PhD
and
Bob Sunberg, MEd

Older adults with low vision sometimes hesitate to go outdoors because of anxiety about traveling by themselves. Add inclement weather and the fear of being identified as a crime target because of an obvious vision problem, and we have a setting where people no longer go outdoors.

For most people, shopping and attending to the tasks of daily living require outdoor travel, as does a visit to the doctor's office or clinic. Most older adults with low vision also wish to continue involvement in recreational and social activities. Regardless of these specific objectives, it is critical for the health of elderly persons to be outdoors and enjoy free movement that contributes to physical health and social interaction. One popular solution for many people is to go to a local mall, where walking clubs and health fairs offer social opportunities of a wide variety.

Within the individual's own turf, some modifications can prevent untoward accidents:

- Wear sunglasses, hats, or visors to shade the eyes and ease the accommodation to bright light.

- Additional lighting, such as a halogen flashlight, may simplify access into the home at night.

Urban dwellers need to learn how to maneuver along busy sidewalks populated by children on skateboards, messengers on bicycles, delivery persons with carts, and pedestrians. Mobility training to help people with low vision use their full complement of senses to maneuver safely is particularly important.

Some problems that can pose threats to safety in rural areas include:

- Unleashed pets and stray animals;.

- Dropoffs of terrain; or

- Absence of paved roads or safe places to walk.

While it would be ideal to construct fences to keep out animals and put up warning signs on sidewalks and highways, the practical solution for the patient with low vision is mobility training.

Orientation and Mobility Instruction

An older adult with vision impairment can often benefit from the services of an Orientation and Mobility specialist, who has received education at the bachelor's or master's level in teaching the visually impaired person to travel independently. Services in orientation and mobility for the visually impaired older individual can often be arranged through the State Vocational Rehabilitation Program that serves blind and visually impaired individuals. In some states, this is an independent commission or bureau, whereas in other states, it is part of the larger, general state rehabilitation program. Private agencies serving persons with visual impairment also provide orientation and mobility services.

The Orientation and Mobility specialist analyzes customary routes with the individual with visual impairment as well as conducting the specialized type of training that enables the person to continue traveling to other places. Realistic orientation and mobility goals are based to some extent upon the person's objectives and an evaluation of the environment. Although many individuals who lose their vision can regain their active lifestyles, others must accept a limitation of activities, because of health, stamina, cognitive ability, or motivation.

Some helpful aids include:

- Low-vision training for the outdoors;
- Distance vision optical aids;
- Prescription cane; or
- Sunwear to reduce glare or increase contrast.

In addition, patients may be interested in contacting clubs and associations that could support their desire to be physically active outdoors.

Transportation

Driving hazards for the patient with vision impairment are well known. Dusk, inclement weather, and tunnels all present risks. The individual may need to be advised to consider alternative transportation, such as buses, paratransit vans, or taxis. Another valuable resource is a neighbor or retiree who may be happy to assist with transportation.

Wherever possible, every effort should be made to encourage the individual with low vision to try to maintain some level of activity and not let vision loss be an overwhelming experience.

Suggested Reading: For Independent Study

Faye EE (ed). *Clinical Low Vision,* 2nd ed. Boston: Little, Brown and Company, 1984.

Freeman PB, Jose R. *The Art and Practice of Low Vision.* Boston: Butterworth-Heinemann, 1991.

Jose RT. *Understanding Low Vision.* New York: American Foundation for the Blind, 1983.

Ophthalmology Study Guide for Students and Practitioners of Medicine, 4th ed. San Francisco: American Academy of Ophthalmology, 1982.

Robrason RG, Robins PV (eds). *Aging and Clinical Practice: Depression and Coexisting Disease.* New York: Igaku-Shoin, 1989.

Rosenthal BP, Cole RG (eds). *A Structured Approach to Low Vision Care. Problems in Optometry.* Vol. 3, no. 3. Philadelphia: J.B. Lippincott, 1991.

Rossman I (ed). *Clinical Geriatrics,* 3rd ed. Philadelphia: J.B. Lippincott, 1986.

Rossman I. The geriatrician and the homebound patient. *J Amer Geriatr Soc* 1988; 36:348-354.

Information and Resource Service

Anyone may call the Lighthouse National Center for Vision and Aging's nationwide toll-free number 800-334-5497 to learn about:

- Age-related eye disorders

- Vision rehabilitation services, including low-vision clinics and training for independent living, and how to locate such services throughout the United States

- Self-help groups for people with visual impairments